I believe this study has great potential in helping Bible
believing people discover the urgency of applying the principles
of Christ to our current challenges of HIV/AIDS. Some of us
were early victims of a fear created by this new disease and the
shame associated with its connection with sexual behavior. I
hope that our number will be greatly diminished by efforts to
see this disease in the context of the love of Christ for the lepers
of His day. The "Burden of a Secret" which I titled my
description of that ordeal in our family, will be lifted if people
have the opportunity to do this kind of study.

– Jimmy R. Allen

Former President of the Southern Baptist Convention
Author of *BURDEN OF A SECRET: A STORY OF TRUTH
AND MERCY IN A FAMILY FACED WITH AIDS*

Indeed, it is time to talk in our churches about HIV and AIDS.
This Bible study discussion guide brings the issue to light in
conversation with some of the Bible's most compelling stories.

– Cheryl J. Sanders

Senior Pastor, Third Street Church of God
Professor of Christian Ethics
Howard University School of Divinity

These timely, well-written and easy to lead lessons guide
without preaching. They combine biblical reference with
personal experience and hope.

– Joan Haner

Member of a women's Bible study group

Time to Talk

in Church

about

HIV and AIDS

A Bible Study Discussion Guide

by

Andrea Bakke and Corean Bakke

Published by

Bakken Books

Acme, Washington

This book is intended to facilitate discussion on the topic of HIV/AIDS and the Church and to provide information on those same topics. The authors developed this book to be a guide to facilitate discussion and not as a medical guide. Care has been taken to provide accurate medical information, yet neither author is a medical doctor, and as such, the authors encourage all readers to seek medical guidance from a trained medical professional for answers to their medical inquires. The authors make no representations beyond the stated intent of this book.

Published by
Bakken Books
PO Box 157, Acme, WA 98220
www.bakkenbooks.com

Scripture quotations are taken from
THE HOLY BIBLE, CONTEMPORARY ENGLISH VERSION
Copyright © 1995 by the American Bible Society
and
THE HOLY BIBLE, AUTHORIZED KING JAMES VERSION

ISBN 0-9755345-0-5

Cover design by Greg Pearson
Photos by Corean Bakke

Contents

When Christians gather, they often prefer to leave unpleasant subjects outside the church doors. For many people, sacred space seems better kept for joyful, peaceful subjects. While Sacred Scriptures contain many unpleasant topics, such passages can be retired to obscurity and not used in worship readings. Perhaps these are some of the reasons behind the reluctance to discuss HIV and AIDS in church.

My daughter-in-law, Andrea, and I designed this book to be a Bible study discussion guide. The lessons draw parallels between leprosy and HIV and AIDS, between a much feared, ancient disease and a modern counterpart. The goal is not to locate right answers – there are no right or wrong answers for many of the questions – but to study and discuss.

Leaders need not be intimidated by the omission of special help for them, found at the back in many Bible study guides. Because the focus here is on discussion, the most effective leaders will not necessarily be those with extensive biblical background or with broad medical knowledge and experience. They will be people who can carefully read a story and apply penetrating observations and questions. If you are the leader, your best preparation is to do each lesson in advance and then allow the group to shape the discussion.

These lessons are appropriate for teenagers and all subsequent ages. The simple format – brief introductory paragraphs followed by a story from the Bible, then discussion questions – is easily adaptable to these diverse age groups. Each lesson offers opportunity for sharing personal experiences, dialogue, listening, and learning.

Two different translations of the Bible are used. The stories for each lesson are taken from the Contemporary English Version. It uses modern-day vocabulary, thereby avoiding vague, antiquated language. This translation, prepared for the American Bible Society, dates from 1995.

The promises at the end of each lesson are taken from the Authorized King James Version dating from 1611, prepared at the request of the King of England. Many people have memorized verses from this version of Scripture. It is included, unaltered, as the traditional biblical language of comfort in the English-speaking world.

We chose photographs of children to introduce each lesson – children from Zambia, Egypt, India, Bangladesh, China, and Bali. Our hearts go out to children and people of all ages whose lives are shattered by this disease.

We chose a Belgian chapel in Boma, Democratic Republic of Congo, to symbolize the global Church. In 1976 a Danish doctor working in that country, then known as Zaire, fell sick with a mysterious illness. Six years later, in 1982, the mysterious illness was given a name: acquired immune deficiency syndrome (AIDS). One year later, health scientists isolated the virus. Not until 1987 was it named human immunodeficiency virus (HIV). By then many countries had reported cases of this illness, and in the United States thousands of infected people had died.[1]

For anyone who wants additional information on HIV and AIDS, we recommend that you check web sites and your library. The quantity of resources is too extensive to include in this small book.

This discussion is for those grieving the loss of loved ones, those watching as this pandemic unfolds, and those whose lives have not yet been touched by HIV and AIDS.

Andrea and I want to thank the many people who have assisted us in preparing this manuscript. Some read the text and offered their expertise; others formed study groups and worked through the lessons. This discussion guide bears the marks of their insight and suggestions.

Corean Bakke

Introduction

The AIDS pandemic has cut short millions of lives all over the world. More people, including children, are infected each year. The grief within millions of families is overwhelming. Communities have been stretched beyond their ability to bear the burden of caring for one another. Countries face financial devastation resulting from loss of a productive work force. Many people are doing great work to assist and educate those affected, but existing efforts cannot begin to keep up with escalating needs.

As I began searching for more information about people living with HIV and AIDS, God was working in my heart challenging me to reach out in some helping way. I soon learned that Corean also had the desire to get involved. We had many discussions about what we were learning. We asked difficult questions as we attempted to determine how we might respond. How could we reach out in love to comfort the grieving, assist families, help orphans, support caregivers, break down the stigma attached to HIV and AIDS, and encourage the Church?

We decided to focus on encouraging the Church, the Bride of Christ, to reach out in love and wrap nurturing arms around her community. We would try to stimulate conversation in churches about HIV and AIDS.

Corean has provided insightful comments. She has located Scriptures relevant to these crises and asked thoughtful discussion questions. This study guide offers groups a way to begin thinking locally and globally as we work together in the effort to eradicate this disease. I pray these lessons will touch you with the love and healing power of Jesus Christ.

Andrea Bakke

HIV: human immunodeficiency virus.

People who are HIV positive are infected with the human immunodeficiency virus. HIV causes disease by multiplying within the white blood cells and attacking the lymphocyte cells that help protect against infection. Significant progress has been made in the treatment of HIV infection. Correct treatments may induce prolonged remission but are not a cure. The virus remains in the body.

HIV is transmitted person-to-person through blood (including menstrual blood), semen, vaginal fluids, and breast milk. The most common ways by which HIV is spread are:

1. Exchange of sexual fluids, semen or vaginal.
2. Blood-to-blood through injections with infected needles and through infusions of infected blood.
3. Mother-to-child through pregnancy (in-utero), childbirth, and breast milk.[2]

Heterosexual contact is the mode of transmission most responsible for the global spread of the virus.

In an HIV infected person, saliva, tears, and feces may contain low numbers of the virus. Transmission is highly unlikely from these body products. Urine contains none.[3]

The virus is not transmitted through casual social contact such as the sharing of eating utensils, the sharing of toilets, shaking hands, hugging, and kissing.[4]

AIDS: acquired immune deficiency syndrome.

People who have AIDS are now in the last stages of HIV infection. The disease has progressed to cause extensive damage to their immune systems. They have become vulnerable to harmful, life threatening infections and complications.

Eventually their body systems become overwhelmed and can no longer continue to function.

If people with AIDS begin prescribed medical treatment, they frequently get better. Badly damaged immune systems can often be greatly improved with proper nourishment and medication.

Syndrome: a collection of symptoms.

Leprosy: an infectious disease caused by the organism *Mycobacterium leprae.*

Not until 1873 was the cause of leprosy known. The Norwegian physician, G.H. Hansen, discovered the organism and subsequently the disease is also known as Hansen's disease.

Since ancient times lepers have been outcasts. Blindness, open sores, and deformities of the nose, hands, and feet commonly result from contracting the disease.

Leprosy is a relatively noninfectious disease. It rarely spreads from person to person. Modern-day treatment does not require isolation.

Leprosy is not hereditary. It is not transmitted through sexual activity nor by food, water, or insects.

It takes a susceptible person and prolonged, close contact to pass the organism. Under these conditions and over a long period of time, the organism can be spread from person to person through infectious nasal discharges and intimate skin contact.

Prolonged treatment with antibiotics effectively kills the organism. Reconstructive plastic surgery can alleviate many of the deformities that develop in neglected cases.

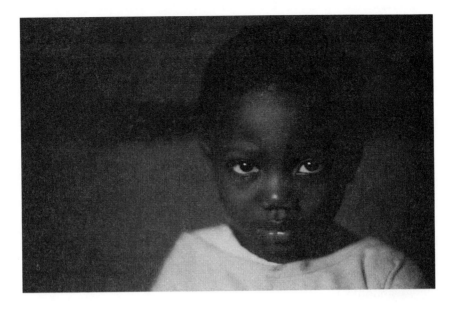

Lesson One

Dreaded Disease in Society

To those living in Bible times, the most dreaded stigma imaginable was to bear the physical signs of leprosy. It totally changed a person's life. No longer permitted to remain within the family and barred from the community, lepers were forced to live outside the city gates, isolated from the healthy populace. Life became a living hell. Deprived of shelter, food, and human relationships, lepers attempted to survive by sorting through garbage for scraps to eat and materials to construct shelters, competing with dogs and other scavengers. The resulting emotional and psychological horrors can only be imagined.

Today infection with HIV has similar effects. A positive diagnosis dramatically changes a person's life. The date becomes a turning point, a grim anniversary of what lies ahead. When medication is available and affordable, the grimness is thrust into the future. When medication is not an option, leaders die young, abandoning society to the elderly and the children. Life for everyone becomes grim.

Leprosy is now understood and has been nearly eradicated from the world. Fewer and fewer people contract the disease and for those who do, treatment is available. In contrast HIV, the virus that causes AIDS, is understood to be one of the most appalling viruses ever observed. Its capacity for reproduction and destruction within the body is nearly unfathomable. And to intensify the misery, death comes slowly. The advance of the virus into healthy populations continues at alarming rates. In terms of the number of people who have died and who will die, it is the worst epidemic in the history of the world. It is truly a monstrous disease and bears its own stigma.

Leprosy in Bible Times

Leviticus 13:1-3, 45-46; 14:1-7

The LORD told Moses and Aaron to say to the people:

If sores or boils or a skin rash should break out and start spreading on your body, you must be brought to Aaron or to one of the other priests. If the priest discovers that the hair in the infected area has turned white and that the infection seems more than skin deep, he will say, "This is leprosy – you are unclean."

If you ever have leprosy, you must tear your clothes, leave your hair uncombed, cover the lower part of your face, and go around shouting, "I'm unclean! I'm unclean!" As long as you have the disease, you are unclean and must live alone outside the camp.

The LORD told Moses to say to the people:

After you think you are healed of leprosy, you must ask for a priest to come outside the camp and examine you. And if you are well, he will have someone bring out two live birds that are acceptable for sacrifice, together with a stick of cedar wood, a piece of red yarn, and a branch from a hyssop plant. The priest will have someone kill one of the birds over a clay pot of spring water. Then he will dip the other bird, the cedar, the red yarn, and the hyssop in the

blood of the dead bird. Next, he will sprinkle you seven
times with the blood and say, "You are now clean."
Finally, he will release the bird and let it fly away.

Discussion Questions

1. What physical conditions alerted people to the possibility
   that they might have leprosy?

2. Who acted as physicians in that ancient society, examining
   the suspicious signs?

3. Describe the diagnosis used to determine leprosy.

4. What were lepers required to do after the diagnosis was confirmed?

5. When lepers thought they were healed, what were they required to do?

6. What words were used to indicate presence of the disease? To indicate absence of the disease?

7. Try to imagine yourself as a person with leprosy. How would you cope?

8. What parallels in diagnosis, treatment, and attitudes do you see between this ancient disease and HIV and AIDS?

9. What are the differences?

10. What are some of the emotional, psychological, and spiritual struggles for people who are HIV positive or have AIDS?

11. In modern society, where physicians examine and diagnose, is there a role for pastors and priests in the AIDS pandemic? If so, what can they do?

It is of the LORD'S mercies

That we are not consumed,

Because his compassions fail not.

They are new every morning:

Great is thy faithfulness.

Lamentations 3:22-23

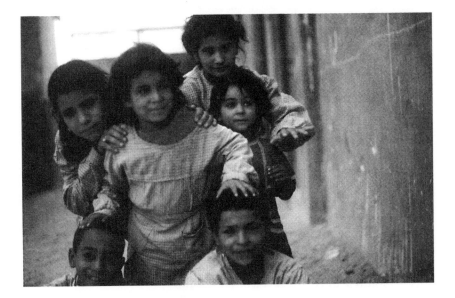

Lesson Two

Contacts with Diseased People

People in Bible times who had leprosy were banished to live outside the city gates. That inhospitable and unsafe place was where the city disposed of everything undesirable: garbage, dogs who ate from it, and the lepers. Those disposed-of-people were required to warn others making their way in or out of the city by calling, "Unclean! Unclean!" Because the disease was not understood, nor was its method of transmission understood, healthy people stayed far away in order to protect themselves.

Many people with HIV and AIDS have experienced banishment from jobs, schools, churches, and family life. They often choose to hide their illness rather than risk the negative and hostile reactions of uninformed and fearful persons afraid to even touch them in simple gestures of friendship. Although people with HIV and AIDS are not banished outside city walls as were their counterparts in Bible times, the personal isolation that occurs when relationships change for the worse is nevertheless stressful and emotionally devastating.

Jesus Heals a Man with Leprosy

Luke 5:12-15

Jesus came to a town where there was a man who had leprosy. When the man saw Jesus, he knelt down to the ground in front of Jesus and begged, "Lord, you have the power to make me well, if only you wanted to."

Jesus put his hand on him and said, "I want to! Now you are well." At once the man's leprosy disappeared. Jesus told him, "Don't tell anyone about this, but go and show yourself to the priest. Offer a gift to the priest, just as Moses commanded and everyone will know that you have been healed."

News about Jesus kept spreading. Large crowds came to listen to him teach and to be healed of their diseases. But Jesus would often go to some place where he could be alone and pray.

Discussion Questions

1. How did the leper in this story fit into the assigned social status given to people with leprosy?

2. Why do you think this leper was so bold?

3. What did Jesus do? What did Jesus say?

4. How did Jewish laws about disease and healing enter into this story?

5. Why would Jesus ask the man to keep silent about his healing?

6. Do you personally know anyone with HIV or AIDS?

7. Did others tell you or were you informed directly by the infected person?

8. How has the disease changed this person?

9. Have HIV and AIDS brought any changes into your life?

10. Do you talk about HIV and AIDS? If so, with whom do you talk?

11. If you do not talk about HIV and AIDS, what are your reasons for keeping silent?

For I am persuaded,

That neither death, nor life,

Nor angels, nor principalities, nor powers,

Nor things present, nor things to come,

Nor height, nor depth,

Nor any other creature,

Shall be able to separate us

From the love of God,

Which is in Christ Jesus our Lord.

Romans 8:38-39

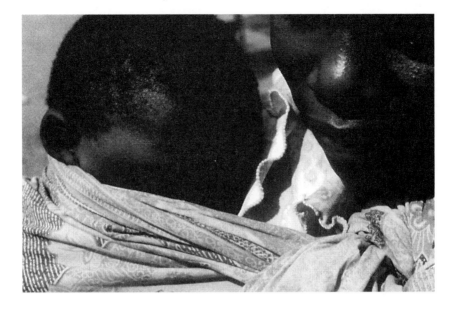

Lesson Three

When HIV and AIDS Come to Church

The first believers were Jews. They had many rules governing their lives. Jesus often puzzled his followers by not conforming to the established rules. When he left them in charge of spreading the Gospel and instructing the next wave of believers, unexpected challenges emerged. Peter's vision on the roof top shocked him into realizing that it was time to set aside rules against associating with Gentiles. This story shows how Peter is pushed out of his comfort zone.

The Church often does not feel comfortable about discussing sex and related topics. Faced with a disease that is transmitted largely through sexual contact, the Church struggles to put human need ahead of moral judgment. Cultures around the world add additional prohibitions to further complicate the problem. It becomes easier to ignore rather than to engage. It becomes easier to hope – and pray – that someone else will step up and relieve the Church of having to take leadership in acting compassionately toward people infected with HIV and AIDS.

23

Instructions to Peter

Acts 10:1-36

In Caesarea there was a man named Cornelius, who was the captain of a group of soldiers called "The Italian Unit." Cornelius was a very religious man. He worshiped God, and so did everyone else who lived in his house. He had given a lot of money to the poor and was always praying to God.

One afternoon at about three o'clock, Cornelius had a vision. He saw an angel from God coming to him and calling him by name. Cornelius was surprised and stared at the angel. Then he asked, "What is this all about?"

The angel answered, "God has heard your prayers and knows about your gifts to the poor. Now send some men to Joppa for a man named Simon Peter. He is visiting with Simon the leather maker, who lives in a house near the sea." After saying this, the angel left.

Cornelius called in two of his servants and one of his soldiers who worshiped God. He explained everything to them and sent them off to Joppa.

The next day about noon these men were coming near Joppa. Peter went up on the roof of the house to pray and became very hungry. While the food was being prepared, he fell sound asleep and had a vision. He saw heaven open, and something came down like a huge sheet held up by its four corners. In it were all kinds of animals, snakes, and birds. A voice said to him, "Peter, get up! Kill these and eat them."

But Peter said, "Lord, I can't do that! I've never eaten anything that is unclean and not fit to eat."

The voice spoke to him again, "When God says that something can be used for food, don't say it isn't fit to eat."

This happened three times before the sheet was suddenly taken back to heaven.

Peter was still wondering what all of this meant, when the men sent by Cornelius came and stood at the gate. They had found their way to Simon's house and were asking if Simon Peter was staying there.

While Peter was still thinking about the vision, the Holy Spirit said to him, "Three men are here looking for you. Hurry down and go with them. Don't worry, I sent them."

Peter went down and said to the men, "I am the one you are looking for. Why have you come?"

They answered, "Captain Cornelius sent us. He is a good man who worships God and is liked by the Jewish people. One of God's holy angels told Cornelius to send for you so he could hear what you have to say." Peter invited them to spend the night.

The next morning, Peter and some of the Lord's followers in Joppa left with the men who had come from Cornelius. The next day they arrived in Caesarea where Cornelius was waiting for them. He had also invited his relatives and close friends.

When Peter arrived, Cornelius greeted him. Then he knelt at Peter's feet and started worshiping him. But Peter took hold of him and said, "Stand up! I am nothing more than a human."

As Peter entered the house, he was still talking with Cornelius. Many people were there, and Peter said to them, "You know that we Jews are not allowed to have anything to do with other people. But God has shown me that he doesn't think anyone is unclean or unfit. I agreed to come here, but I want to know why you sent for me."

Cornelius answered:

Four days ago at about three o'clock in the afternoon I was praying at home. Suddenly a man in bright clothes stood in front of me. He said, "Cornelius, God has heard your prayers, and he knows about your gifts to the poor. Now send to Joppa for Simon Peter. He is visiting in the home of Simon the leather maker, who lives near the sea."

I sent for you right away, and you have been good enough to come. All of us are here in the presence of the Lord God, so that we can hear what he has to say.

Peter then said:

Now I am certain that God treats all people alike. God is pleased with everyone who worships him and does right, no matter what nation they come from. This is the same message that God gave to the people of Israel, when he sent Jesus Christ, the Lord of all, to offer peace to them.

Discussion Questions

1. What had Peter been accustomed to eating? Leviticus 11 lists the animals that the Jewish people could eat and those that they were not to eat.

2. Identify the forbidden animals presented to Peter in this vision.

3. What was Peter's response when told to kill and eat?

4. What was God's response to hearing Peter's declaration of eating by the rules?

5. Describe the events and the timing of events following each vision.

6. Have you ever been pushed out of your comfort zone? How did it happen? In what ways has your life been different since then?

7. You may have been part of a church that had to face new and uncomfortable realities. Describe that experience.

8. Are HIV and AIDS talked about in your church? If they are, how?

9. How are people living with HIV and AIDS talked about and treated in your church?

10. Do you see any way to connect this story about Peter with HIV and AIDS?

And I will bring the blind

By a way that they knew not;

I will lead them in paths that they have not known:

I will make darkness light before them,

And crooked things straight.

These things will I do unto them,

And not forsake them.

Isaiah 42:16

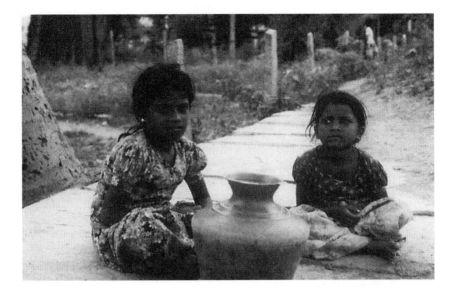

Lesson Four

HIV and AIDS at the Communion Table

Unlike Moslems, Hindus, and Jews, Christians eat and drink during worship in a ritual of sharing. Many churches continue to practice common cup, the ancient tradition whereby everyone drinks from the same chalice. When it was discovered that invisible organisms cause the spread of countless diseases, the practice of using individual cups at communion emerged. As a result, many churches serve communion wine in tiny cups, one for each person, so that no one runs the risk of ingesting germs. The possible presence of people with HIV and AIDS at the communion table has alerted manufacturers of tiny, individual plastic cups to intensify their advertising. They point out the desirability of their product in this climate of fear with the slogan, "Better safe than sorry."

Two statements bear repeating here in view of unsupportable yet persistent fear at the communion table. Sensing his visitors' jitters over the prospect of communing from a common cup along with dirty and unkempt people in the cathedral, a Bishop in Pakistan explained: "No one gets sick drinking the blood of our Lord."

31

The second is a cryptic, cynical comment of exasperation over ignorance in the church. "The only way to get AIDS at communion is to have unprotected sex with an HIV positive person either before or after communion."

The story of Jesus at the home of Simon focuses attention on the problem of hospitality toward people with dreaded diseases. Simon had leprosy. Instead of finding Simon outside the city gates shouting, "Unclean, unclean!" we find him hosting a dinner party. There is much here to wonder about.

Jesus at the Home of Simon

Matthew 26:6-13

Jesus was in the town of Bethany, eating at the home of Simon, who had leprosy. A woman came in with a bottle of expensive perfume and poured it on Jesus' head. But when his disciples saw this, they became angry and complained, "Why such a waste? We could have sold this perfume for a lot of money and given it to the poor."

Jesus knew what they were thinking, and he said:

Why are you bothering this woman? She has done a beautiful thing for me. You will always have the poor with you, but you won't always have me. She has poured perfume on my body to prepare it for burial. You may be sure that wherever the good news is told all over the world, people will remember what she has done. And they will tell others.

Discussion Questions

1. What was Jesus doing at Simon's house?

2. Was there any prohibition against healthy people eating with lepers in Bible times?

3. Why would Simon invite Jesus to his home for a meal?

4. Was Jesus the only guest at Simon's table? What other people are mentioned in the story?

5. The story reveals a crisis during the meal. Describe what happened.

6. The host's disease is not the focus of the story. It seems to be included to identify Simon. Why do you think leprosy in this story was treated so casually?

7. Would you invite a person who is infected with HIV to your home for dinner?

8. At the communion table in your church how is the wine served? Why?

9. Would you be afraid of sharing common cup with a person you knew to be infected with HIV?

10. Would you be afraid of sharing common cup with a person you knew to have AIDS?

11. How do you think persons with HIV and AIDS might feel if they observed cautious behavior at communion?

For ye shall go out with joy,

And be led forth with peace:

The mountains and the hills

Shall break forth before you into singing,

And all the trees of the field

Shall clap their hands.

Isaiah 55:12

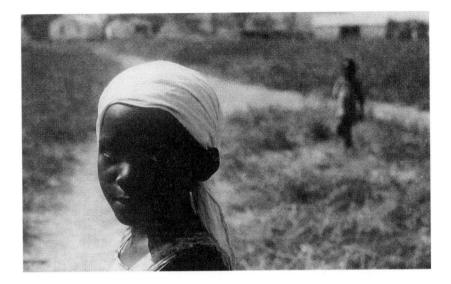

Lesson Five

Living with HIV and AIDS

This story began in Syria, a country with its own public health policies. Naaman, infected with leprosy, continued to work. He had not been forced to quit his job. His boss respected him. His family and servants supported him.

People living with HIV and AIDS often choose to keep their diagnosis secret. Informing others jeopardizes their employment, their social life, and their family life. The sum total of their lives is affected from the day of diagnosis. They are very vulnerable. They struggle with disbelief, anger, and depression as they try to absorb the reality of what has happened to them. Things said and done at this time can easily hurt them. They need people with whom they can feel safe and places where they can feel safe. They very often have neither.

Naaman

2 Kings 5:1-15

Naaman was the commander of the Syrian army. The Lord had helped him and his troops defeat their enemies, so the king of Syria respected Naaman very much. Naaman was a brave soldier, but he had leprosy.

One day while the Syrian troops were raiding Israel, they captured a girl, and she became a servant of Naaman's wife. Some time later the girl said, "If your husband Naaman would go to the prophet in Samaria, he would be cured of his leprosy."

When Naaman told the king what the girl had said, the king replied, "Go ahead! I will give you a letter to take to the king of Israel."

Naaman left and took along seven hundred fifty pounds of silver, one hundred fifty pounds of gold, and ten new outfits. He also carried the letter to the king of Israel. It said, "I am sending my servant Naaman to you. Would you cure him of his leprosy?"

When the king of Israel read the letter, he tore his clothes in fear and shouted, "That Syrian king believes I can cure this man of leprosy! Does he think I'm God with power over life and death? He must be trying to pick a fight with me."

As soon as Elisha the prophet heard what had happened, he sent the Israelite king this message: "Why are you so afraid? Send the man to me, so that he will know there is a prophet in Israel."

Naaman left with his horses and chariots and stopped at the door of Elisha's house. Elisha sent someone outside to say to him, "Go wash seven times in the Jordan River. Then you'll be completely cured."

But Naaman stormed off, grumbling, "Why couldn't he come out and talk to me? I thought for sure he would stand in front of me and pray to the Lord his God, then wave his hand over my skin and cure me. What about the Abana River or the Pharpar River?

Those rivers in Damascus are just as good as any river in Israel. I could have washed in them and been cured."

His servants went over to him and said, "Sir, if the prophet had told you to do something difficult, you would have done it. So why don't you do what he said? Go wash and be cured."

Naaman walked down to the Jordan; he waded out into the water and stooped down in it seven times, just as Elisha had told him. Right away, he was cured, and his skin became as smooth as a child's.

Naaman and his officials went back to Elisha. Naaman stood in front of him and announced; "Now I know that the God of Israel is the only God in the whole world. Sir, would you please accept a gift from me?"

Discussion Questions

1. Explain Naaman's role in Syrian society. What relationship existed between Naaman and the king?

2. The story mentions a military skirmish between Syria and another nation. An incident, common between warring nations, occurred. Describe.

3. This incident took on extraordinary meaning and potential. Explain what happened in Naaman's household.

4. Naaman was desperate to find healing for his leprosy. He had the support of his king and his soldiers, his wife and her servants. But he almost failed in his quest for healing because of a common character trait. Describe.

5. Has any person ever confided to you that she or he is infected with HIV or has AIDS? Why would a person confide this information?

6. What was your response? Were you helpful or were you hurtful? How could a person respond in a helpful way?

7. How did other people respond to that news of infection with HIV?

8. Describe your church. Is it a safe place for persons with HIV and AIDS? Explain.

9. Can you think of ways to enable your church to be a more welcoming and helpful place for people with HIV and AIDS?

A friend loveth at all times,

And a brother is born for adversity.

Proverb 17:17

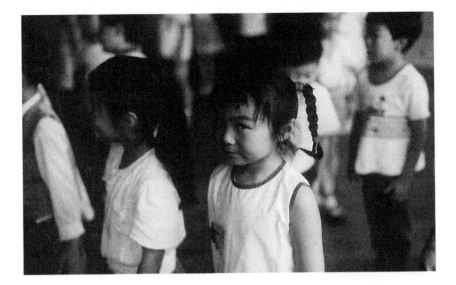

Lesson Six

Dying with AIDS

The story in chapter 26 of 2 Chronicles follows, with much detail, a career begun at age 16. Uzziah seemed to make all the right choices as he energetically and creatively strengthened the Kingdom of Judah. But success made him arrogant and proud. His downfall came swiftly. Leprosy put him out of control and out of the palace. When he died, he could not even be buried in the royal tombs.

AIDS occurs when the HIV multiplies within lymphocytes (white blood cells that fight infection and certain types of cancer) and destroys them. Because of this, people become vulnerable to infection and malignant cells developing within the body. Minor infections, routinely repelled by healthy immune systems, become major illnesses in bodies with crippled and broken-down immune systems. For the same reason, cancers are able to develop and grow unchecked. People with AIDS become seriously ill with multiple infections and/or cancers. Their bodies weaken until they can no longer cope with the many things that are going wrong. Emotionally and spiritually exhausted by efforts to stay alive, they give up. Death comes as a welcome release.

The list of people whose lives have been terminated by AIDS continues to grow. Many of them die in the prime of life, leaving enormous gaps in their professions, families, and communities. This is happening all around the world with frightening speed and with frightening consequences. The sheer volume of funerals in some communities puts hardships on friends and family members who want to pay their last respects, but are unable to give the time their cultures prescribe for final farewells. AIDS is confronting society with many problems.

King Uzziah

2 Chronicles 26

After the death of King Amaziah, the people of Judah crowned his son Uzziah king, even though he was only sixteen at the time. Uzziah ruled fifty-two years from Jerusalem, the hometown of his mother Jecoliah. During his rule, he recaptured and rebuilt the town of Elath.

He obeyed the LORD by doing right, as his father Amaziah had done. Zechariah was Uzziah's advisor and taught him to obey God. And so, as long as Zechariah was alive, Uzziah was faithful to God, and God made him successful.

While Uzziah was king, he started a war against the Philistines. He smashed the walls of the cities of Gath, Jabneh, and Ashdod, then rebuilt towns around Ashdod and in other parts of Philistia. God helped him defeat the Philistines, the Arabs living in Gur-Baal, and the Meunites. Even the Ammonites paid taxes to Uzziah. He became very powerful, and people who lived as far away as Egypt heard about him.

In Jerusalem, Uzziah built fortified towers at the Corner Gate, the Valley Gate, and the place where the city wall turned inward. He also built defense towers out in the desert.

He owned such a large herd of livestock in the western foothills and in the flatlands, that he had cisterns dug there to catch the rainwater. He loved farming, so he had crops and vineyards planted in the hill country wherever there was fertile soil, and he hired farmers to take care of them.

Uzziah's army was always ready for battle. Jeiel and Maaseiah were the officers who kept track of the number of soldiers, all under the command of Hananiah, one of Uzziah's officials. There were 307,500 trained soldiers, all under the command of 2,600 clan leaders. These powerful troops protected the king against any enemy. Uzziah supplied his army with shields, spears, helmets, armor, bows, and stones used for slinging. Some of his skilled workers invented machines that could shoot arrows and sling large stones. Uzziah set these up in Jerusalem at his defense towers and at the corners of the city wall.

God helped Uzziah become more and more powerful, and he was famous all over the world.

Uzziah became proud of his power and this led to his downfall.

One day, Uzziah disobeyed the LORD his God by going into the temple and burning incense as an offering to him. Azariah the priest and eighty other brave priests followed Uzziah into the temple and said, "Your Majesty, this isn't right! You are not allowed to burn incense to the Lord. That must be done only by priests who are descendants of Aaron. You will have to leave! You have sinned against the LORD, and so he will no longer bless you."

Uzziah, who was standing next to the incense altar at the time, was holding the incense burner, ready to offer incense to the Lord. He became very angry when he heard Azariah's warning, and leprosy suddenly appeared on his forehead! Azariah and the other priests saw it and immediately told him to leave the temple. Uzziah realized that the LORD had punished him, so he hurried to get outside.

*Uzziah had leprosy the rest of his life. He was no
longer allowed in the temple or in his own palace.
That's why his son Jotham lived there and ruled in his
place.*

*Everything else Uzziah did while he was king is in
the records written by the prophet Isaiah son of Amoz.
Since Uzziah had leprosy, he could not be buried in the
royal tombs. Instead, he was buried in a nearby
cemetery that the kings owned. His son Jotham then
became king.*

Discussion Questions

1. How long did King Uzziah rule Judah? What age did he
   begin and at what age did he finish?

2. What was the secret of his success? Identify some of his
   successes as king.

3. What did he do that was wrong? Describe the confrontation in the temple.

4. What happened as the result of his doing wrong?

5. Were all cases of leprosy in Bible times consequences of doing wrong?

6. Do you think HIV and AIDS are punishment for doing wrong? Does your church think HIV and AIDS are punishment for doing wrong?

7. Jesus cautioned his followers about judging other people. Read and discuss what Jesus said in Matthew 7:1-6.

8. Dying from multiple illnesses as the result of a no-longer-functioning immune system is slow and painful. Do you have any significant memories to share about this process?

9. How does your thinking about HIV and AIDS affect your attitudes and actions toward people who are dying from multiple illnesses as a result of HIV infection?

10. What is the responsibility of the Church to people who are dying with AIDS? Read and discuss Jesus' words in Matthew 25:31-46.

Blessed are they that mourn:

For they shall be comforted.

Matthew 5:4

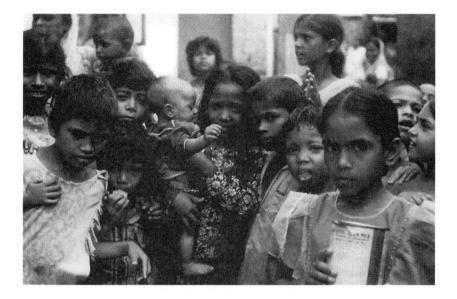

Lesson Seven

Protection from HIV

Jesus turned a massive following into a lesson in responsibility for his disciples. In the face of enormous need and pitiful supplies, Jesus tested the resolve and the resources of his most personal followers.

People who learn about the seriousness of HIV and AIDS are quickly overwhelmed by the need and by the lack of supplies and support systems available to meet that need. People uninformed about the disease cannot assume they will remain unaffected.

HIV is the name of the virus that causes AIDS. Its full name is human immunodeficiency virus. It works by breaking down the natural immune system and making the body vulnerable to endless and multiple illnesses until, finally, the body cannot function any longer. Death comes slowly and painfully.

HIV is transmitted by body fluid contact with a person who already has the virus. The infected person may be unaware of having it and may appear to be perfectly healthy. Not until the immune system begins to break down, is there any hint of having the disease.

These are ways HIV is spread:
1. By unprotected vaginal, anal, or oral sex with someone who is infected with HIV
2. By sharing needles with someone who is infected with HIV
3. From an infected mother to her baby during pregnancy, childbirth or breast feeding
4. Infusion of HIV-infected blood
5. Needlestick injuries while caring for infected people
6. Organ transplants from infected donors[5]

Many people do not know how HIV is spread. Because the primary way to get infected is sexual, and because sex is private and not openly discussed, these realities create serious problems. An important first step is simply to end the silence and start talking. Put cultural and religious taboos aside. Be truthful and honest.

Jesus Demonstrates Responsibility for the Entire Community

John 6:1-13

Jesus crossed Lake Galilee, which was also known as Lake Tiberias. A large crowd had seen him work miracles to heal the sick, and those people went with him. It was almost time for the Jewish festival of Passover, and Jesus went up on a mountain with his disciples and sat down.

When Jesus saw the large crowd coming toward him, he asked Philip, "Where will we get enough food to feed all these people?" He said this to test Philip, since he already knew what he was going to do.

Philip answered, "Don't you know that it would take almost a year's wages just to buy only a little bread for each of these people?"

56

Andrew, the brother of Simon Peter, was one of the disciples. He spoke up and said, "There is a boy here who has five small loaves of barley bread and two fish. But what good is that with all these people?"

The ground was covered with grass, and Jesus told his disciples to have everyone sit down. About five thousand men were in the crowd. Jesus took the bread in his hands and gave thanks to God. Then he passed the bread to the people, and he did the same with the fish, until everyone had plenty to eat.

The people ate all they wanted, and Jesus told his disciples to gather up the leftovers, so that nothing would be wasted. The disciples gathered them up and filled twelve large baskets with what was left over from the five barley loaves.

Discussion Questions

1. What could the disciples have been thinking when they saw the crowds of hungry people?

2. How did Philip respond to Jesus' question?

3. What was Andrew's simple response to Jesus' question?

4. What answer could Jesus have been seeking?

5. When looking at HIV and AIDS worldwide, we see a nearly hopeless situation. Is there a simple solution? Explain.

6. HIV is now a universal health crisis. How can people in your community become informed about the spread and prevention of this disease?

7. What information do people need? Who should be responsible for providing information?

8. What customs and behaviors put people at risk for sexually transmitted HIV?

9. In cultures where women are subject to men, who needs to take responsibility for protecting young girls and women from HIV?

10. In order to reduce the number of people becoming infected with HIV, some kind of prevention program must be implemented. What could be a responsible prevention program for your community?

11. Should leaders of church and community be publicly responsible for their sexual practices? Why or why not? If yes, how?

12. Churches have the potential to become change agents in their communities. How is your church participating in HIV prevention programs?

13. What is the relationship between this story from Scripture and protection from HIV?

The LORD is righteous in all his ways,

And holy in all his works.

The LORD is nigh unto all them that call upon him,

To all that call upon him in truth.

He will fulfill the desire of them that fear him:

He also will hear their cry,

And will save them.

Psalm 145:17-19

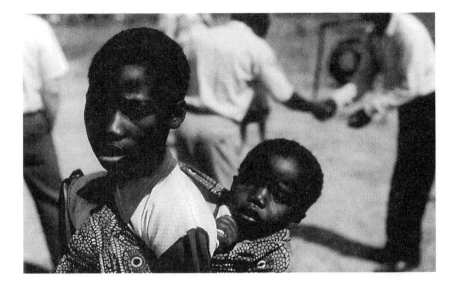

Lesson Eight

The Changing Family

Jesus, as the first-born son, had the responsibility of caring for his mother. She watched as he hung dying on the cross. From that public place of shame, he made provision for her by asking John, his favorite disciple, to adopt her as his mother and by asking Mary to adopt John as her son.

HIV and AIDS are making millions of children orphans. On the continent of Africa, where extended families are legendary, onlookers supposed that abandoned children would be automatically absorbed into the caring protection of aunts, uncles, and grandparents. But the stigma of HIV and AIDS carries over to the children who are left behind. They are not wanted. They might contaminate others. Where homes are open to them, the steadily increasing burden of care for dependent children threatens to exhaust capabilities. As a result, children are forced to take responsibility for younger siblings, living as best they can separately from adults. This dilemma is beyond comprehension. Entire communities totter on the brink of chaos.

Jesus Restructures His Family

John 19:16b-27

Jesus was taken away, and he carried his cross to a place known as "The Skull." In Aramaic this place is called "Golgotha." There Jesus was nailed to the cross, and on each side of him a man was also nailed to a cross.

Pilate ordered the charge against Jesus to be written on a board and put above the cross. It read, "Jesus of Nazareth, King of the Jews." The words were written in Hebrew, Latin, and Greek.

The place where Jesus was taken wasn't far from the city, and many of the people read the charge against him. So the chief priests went to Pilate and said, "Why did you write that he is King of the Jews? You should have written, 'He claimed to be King of the Jews.'"

But Pilate told them, "What is written will not be changed!"

After the soldiers had nailed Jesus to the cross, they divided up his clothes into four parts, one for each of them. But his outer garment was made from a single piece of cloth, and it did not have any seams. The soldiers said to each other, "Let's not rip it apart. We will gamble to see who gets it." This happened so that the Scriptures would come true, which say, "They divided up my clothes and gambled for my garments." The soldiers then did what they had decided.

Jesus' mother stood beside his cross with her sister and Mary the wife of Clopas. Mary Magdalene was standing there too. When Jesus saw his mother and his favorite disciple with her, he said to his mother, "This man is now your son." Then he said to the disciple, "She is now your mother." From then on, that disciple took her into his own home.

Discussion Questions

1. From your reading of Bible stories, what family structures have you found? The books of Genesis, Ruth, 1 and 2 Samuel contain most of the stories about families.

2. What position did a first-born son have in the Bible time family? What were his responsibilities?

3. As Jesus was dying, he chose John to provide for his mother. Were there others who could have provided for Mary? Read and discuss Mark 6:1-6.

4. Why did Jesus choose John? Read and discuss Mark 3:31-35.

5. How do you think Mary would have survived following Jesus' death if she had not gone to live with John?

6. In times of shock or need, what changes in family structures may occur?

7. How can extended families be assisted as they attempt to cope with the sudden increase of children orphaned by AIDS?

8. Orphanages have been established in many countries, often by outside agencies. Is this a good solution to caring for children without parents? Read and discuss James 1:27.

9. Today, prospective parents may travel halfway around the world to adopt children. This means that children are removed from their country and their culture. Is this a good solution?

10. What other interventions could be considered as a solution to caring for children orphaned by AIDS?

11. It will take many creative ideas and enormous energy to make a difference in the lives of orphans. Do you have any ideas for bringing hope to this huge dilemma?

Hast thou not known? Hast thou not heard,

That the everlasting God,

The LORD, the Creator of the ends of the earth,

Fainteth not, neither is weary?

There is no searching of his understanding.

He giveth power to the faint;

And to them that have no might he increaseth strength.

Even the youths shall faint and be weary,

And the young men shall utterly fall:

But they that wait upon the LORD shall renew their strength;

They shall mount up with wings as eagles;

They shall run, and not be weary;

And they shall walk, and not faint.

Isaiah 40:28-31

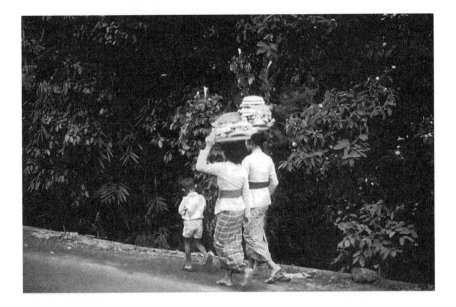

Lesson Nine

Care Giving

Jesus told a story to illustrate genuine concern for needy people. The story included a severely injured man and three potential caregivers. Two of them were religious people. The third was described only by his ethnic identity, one that placed him in the underclass of Jewish society. The religious people chose not to get involved. The person of low status interrupted his plans and took care of the injured man. This story of compassion has touched the hearts of people for centuries.

Religious leaders have been noticeably absent from the ranks of those caring for people with HIV and AIDS. Preaching, teaching, and evangelistic zeal provide focus for ministry in directions that often avoid meeting the physical needs of people. Pastors, priests, seminary professors, Bible teachers, mission executives, and their respective organizations many times fail to appear on the lists of community groups involved with people ill and dying with HIV and AIDS. Their reasons for avoiding involvement may resemble those of the religious people in Jesus' story.

Jesus Tells a Parable about Care Giving

Luke 10:25-37

An expert in the Law of Moses stood up and asked Jesus a question to see what he would say. "Teacher," he asked, "what must I do to have eternal life?"

Jesus answered, "What is written in the Scriptures? How do you understand them?"

The man replied, "The Scriptures say, 'Love the Lord your God with all your heart, soul, strength, and mind.' They also say, 'Love your neighbors as much as you love yourself.' "

Jesus said, "You have given the right answer. If you do this, you will have eternal life"

But the man wanted to show that he knew what he was talking about. So he asked Jesus, "Who are my neighbors?"

Jesus replied:

As a man was going down from Jerusalem to Jericho, robbers attacked him and grabbed everything he had. They beat him up and ran off, leaving him half dead.

A priest happened to be going down the same road. But when he saw the man, he walked by on the other side. Later a temple helper came to the same place. But when he saw the man who had been beaten up, he also went by on the other side.

A man from Samaria then came traveling along that road. When he saw the man, he felt sorry for him and went over to him. He treated his wounds with olive oil and wine and bandaged them. Then he put him on his own donkey and took him to an inn, where he took care of him. The next morning he gave the innkeeper two silver coins and said, "Please take care of the man. If you spend more than this on him, I will pay you when I return."

Then Jesus asked, "Which one of these three people was a real neighbor to the man who was beaten up by robbers?"

The teacher answered, "The one who showed pity."

Jesus said, "Go and do the same!"

Discussion Questions

1. In the story, how did the religious men know that the victim needed help?

2. Why do you think they chose not to get involved?

3. Why do you think the Samaritan stopped to help?

4. If the man lying half-dead on the road was a Jew, the Samaritan's efforts to give assistance might go unappreciated. Why?

5. How did the Samaritan help?

6. The next morning at the inn, the story focused on three people. Who were they and what were they doing?

7. What are some of the needs of a person with AIDS? How could a caregiver provide assistance?

8. Have you ever been a caregiver or known someone who was?

9. If, as in the story, two out of three people choose not to get involved, this places a heavy burden on the one who does. How does a caregiver wear out?

10. Did the story model any guidelines for giving help while at the same time protecting resources?

11. When caregivers come to the end of their resources, especially their emotional resources, and the need to care remains, what could they do?

12. Does your church recognize caregivers as people with names and needs or are they seen as extensions of the wheelchairs they push? What is the role of churches in recognizing and supporting caregivers?

Come unto me,

All ye that labor and are heavy laden,

And I will give you rest.

Take my yoke upon you,

And learn of me;

For I am meek and lowly in heart:

And ye shall find rest unto your souls.

For my yoke is easy,

And my burden is light.

Matthew 11:28-30

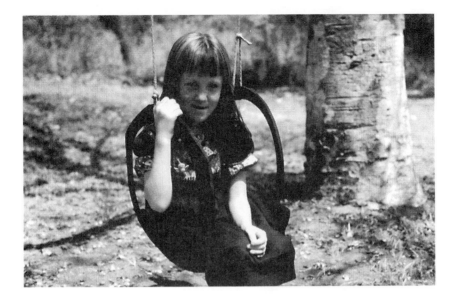

Lesson Ten

The Promise

The disciples came to realize that Jesus spent considerable time praying. They heard him pray. They watched him pray. They waited for him to return from his private prayers. Realizing how important prayer was to Jesus, the disciples requested a lesson in how to pray. The model prayer that Jesus gave them is now known as the Lord's Prayer. His prayer instruction continued. The disciples were charged to be aggressive in their prayers and not give up. The answer to a prayer of asking is receiving. The answer to a prayer about searching is finding. The answer to a prayer about knocking is an opened door.

HIV and AIDS are making life grim and hopeless beyond imagination for many people throughout the world. This disease is cutting a wide swath of debilitation and death through the heart of populations, leaving only the young and the old behind. Aging grandmothers are inheriting sole responsibility for numerous grandchildren. Unemployed themselves, and usually without resources, these women must feed, clothe, house, and educate the orphaned children of their sons and daughters.

Custom will not soon change in areas of the world where laws deny status and self-determination to women and give rights of land and property to men. Yet the women, those most vulnerable and least protected, must shoulder the horrendous burden of providing everything out of nothing.

Jesus Teaches His Disciples How to Pray

Luke 11:1-13

When Jesus had finished praying, one of his disciples said to him, "Lord, teach us to pray, just as John taught his followers to pray."

So Jesus told them, "Pray in this way:

'Father, help us to honor your name. Come and set up your kingdom. Give us each day the food we need. Forgive our sins, as we forgive everyone who has done wrong to us. And keep us from being tempted.'"

Then Jesus went on to say:

Suppose one of you goes to a friend in the middle of the night and says, "Let me borrow three loaves of bread. A friend of mine has dropped in, and I don't have a thing for him to eat." And suppose your friend answers, "Don't bother me! The door is bolted, and my children and I are in bed. I cannot get up to give you something."

He may not get up and give you the bread, just because you are his friend. But he will get up and give you as much as you need, simply because you are not ashamed to keep on asking.

So I tell you to ask and you will receive, search and you will find, knock and the door will be opened for you. Everyone who asks will receive, everyone who searches will find, and the door will be opened for everyone who knocks. Which one of you fathers would give your hungry child a snake if the child asks for a fish? Which one of you would give your child a scorpion if the child asked for an egg? As bad as you are, you still know how to give good gifts to your children. But your heavenly Father is even more ready to give the Holy Spirit to anyone who asks.

Discussion Questions

1. Jesus gave his disciples a model prayer known as the Lord's Prayer. Based on this model what should prayer include?

2. What things does Jesus teach us to ask for ourselves?

3. How did Jesus use food to expand his teaching on prayer?

4. In this teaching on prayer, what point is Jesus making when he contrasts bad gifts with good gifts?

5. Why is prayer an important practice in the HIV and AIDS pandemic?

6. Does God answer prayers through the efforts and creativity of friends and acquaintances? Can you name some examples of answered prayers?

7. Does God answer prayers through the efforts of the Church? Can you name some examples?

8. Why does Jesus name the Holy Spirit as the best gift of all?

9. How do you think the Holy Spirit brings answers to the prayers of people and communities devastated by HIV and AIDS?

Therefore take no thought, saying,

What shall we eat? or,

What shall we drink? or,

Wherewithal shall we be clothed?

(For after all these things do the Gentiles seek:)

For your heavenly Father knoweth

That ye have need of all these things.

But seek ye first the kingdom of God,

And his righteousness;

And all these things shall be added unto you.

Matthew 6:31-33

Afterword

As I write this concluding page, I am still learning about HIV and AIDS.

My first encounter occurred in the spring of 1990. I was a student at Chicago Theological Seminary and enrolled in a course titled "Pastoral Care in the Church." A guest lecturer described her involvement in a unique ministry: AIDS Pastoral Care Network. She directed pastoral services and trained volunteers. I became a volunteer.

Three years later a friend died with AIDS. Four years later a friend was diagnosed with HIV. When a leading news magazine published a cover story describing the rapid expansion of AIDS in Africa, Andrea and I decided to write this book. Finally, we are on the last page. My encounter with this disease is in its fourteenth year.

The decision to write a Bible study discussion guide for the Church is audacious and humbling. Our qualifications are slim. How can we be sure that our personal observations carry relevance for others in the Church? Your encounter with HIV and AIDS may be less than ours; however, it may be substantially greater.

Each lesson concludes with an unconditional promise from Scripture, words of hope. These promises stand firm regardless of anything anyone of us might do or fail to do.

Having come to the final page, and now wondering what next step to take, my thoughts turn to Jesus' words in the Sermon on the Mount from Matthew chapter five:

> *You are like salt for everyone on earth. But if salt no longer tastes like salt, how can it make food salty? All it is good for is to be thrown out and walked on.*

You are like light for the whole world. A city built on top of a hill cannot be hidden, and no one would light a lamp and put it under a clay pot. A lamp is placed on a lampstand, where it can give light to everyone in the house. Make your light shine, so that others will see the good that you do and will praise your Father in heaven.

Jesus speaks to me in language I understand when he likens my presence in the world to salt in my kitchen. I could neither bake nor cook without salt. Is my presence that critical to the well-being of my community?

I live in the country. When neither moon nor stars can be seen, thick darkness surrounds me. On such nights, the tiny light on my doorbell shines with amazing brightness, penetrating the outdoor expanse and drawing attention to my front entrance.

Jesus' words – to be as salt and light in my community – become a daily reminder. I wonder what I will encounter next with this modern affliction.

HIV and AIDS present a great challenge to the Church to be as salt and light, to make a difference in people's lives. This opportunity to show compassion to the sick and dying and those left behind has no limits.

As you met with your Bible study discussion group, did you think about getting involved? Pray for guidance. You will find it.

If you wish to tell us about your experience with the book, Andrea and I would be happy to hear from you.

Thank you for joining in this discussion.

Corean Bakke

Final Questions

Now that you have completed these ten lessons, your responses to the following five questions would be very helpful. Please send comments via e-mail to andrea@bakkenbooks.com or mail to Bakken Books, PO Box 157, Acme, WA 98220.

1. Was there anything you did not understand?

2. What was missing?

3. What was not needed?

4. How did you feel these lessons were helpful?

5. Did you have a favorite lesson? What made it special?

Endnotes

1. These dates are taken from the following chronological record of HIV and AIDS beginning in 1976: Randy Shilts, *And the Band Played On: People, Politics, and the AIDS Epidemic*, St. Martin's Press, New York, 1987.

2. John G. Bartlett, M.D., and Ann K. Finkbeiner, *The Guide to Living with HIV Infection,* 5th ed., Johns Hopkins University Press, Baltimore, Md., 2001, p. 33.

3. Ibid, p. 34.

4. Ibid, p. 33.

5. Ibid, pp. 33-34.

About the Authors

Andrea Bakke

Andrea is co-founder with Corean of Bakken Books. She is a member of the board of directors of the Mustard Seed Foundation, a Sunday School teacher, and a Girl Scout leader. She has a BA in Human Relations. Her work experience in Christian ministries includes International Urban Associates (IUA), Chariot Family Publishing, and church secretary. Her interest in serving those affected by HIV and AIDS comes from her foundation work and her role as mother of an African-American child.

Andrea is married to Woody Bakke and they are adoptive parents of two children, Amber and Elijah. They are members of a United Methodist church.

Corean Bakke

Corean is artist-in-residence at Bakken, family home and location of Bakken Books. She has degrees in music and theology. She is a concert pianist and has taught piano at the collegiate level. Her travel experiences include Africa, Asia, the Middle East, and Europe. Corean is a published author with titles including: *Let the Whole World Sing: The Story Behind the Music of Lausanne II,* a narrative of planning worship for an international congress in the Philippines; and, *Aleluya,* an international hymnal produced jointly with Tony Payne. She worked as editor for *Christianity and the Arts*, a quarterly magazine. She learned about AIDS Pastoral Care Network while in seminary and prepared herself for involvement by completing the volunteer training course.

Corean is married to Ray Bakke, mother of three sons, and a grandmother. She is a member of a Lutheran church in Bellingham, Washington.